Ready to Wean

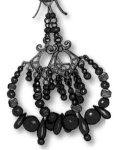

or *The Return
of the Dangling
Red Earrings*

Elyse April

Illustrations by Diane Iverson

Foreword by Deborah Auletta, RN, IBCLC

"To the HOHM Press/ Kalindi Press Staff for all their support and friendship."

© 2012 , Elyse April

Cover illustration: Diane Iverson
Cover Design, Interior Design and Layout: Zac Parker, Kadak Graphics, Prescott, Arizona

Library of Congress Cataloging in Publication Data:

ISBN: 978-1-935387-30-5

Hohm Press
P.O. Box 4410
Chino Valley, AZ 86323
800-381-2700
www.hohmpress.com

Printed in China

FOREWORD

The American Academy of Pediatrics states that women should breastfeed their babies for one year and then until mutually desirable for both parties. The World Health Organization (WHO) says women should breastfeed their babies for two years or longer. Ultimately, however, the choice of when to wean one's child is a very personal one. *Ready to Wean*, the lovely new book from Elyse April and Hohm Press, will leave women feeling supported and empowered in their completion of breastfeeding and through the transition into all the continuing and new ways that mothers and children love one another. The only question remaining for me is why has no one written this book sooner?

—**Deborah Auletta, RN, IBCLC**, co-author of
Breastfeeding: Your Priceless Gift to Your Baby and Yourself

NOTE TO PARENTS

HOW TO EASILY & GENTLY STOP NURSING

The transition from nursing to weaning marks a special time in the development of a baby or child. It can either be a time full of stress, regret and confusion, or a joyous celebration of growth – a movement toward becoming a full and vibrant human being.

This book is for you and your child, to help you both communicate your deep love and respect for one another. I believe that it is never too early to talk to your baby with tenderness and dignity, and to explain that nursing together is a cherished and special time. Yet, when mother no longer chooses this mutual task, or for health or other reasons cannot continue, then it is better for parent and child to begin weaning. Here are a few suggestions to help make this an easy and gentle process.

1. PREPARE YOUR CHILD. Once you are seriously thinking about weaning, begin talking to your little one about it. Do this at the same time that you are actually nursing and caressing them. Speak of a day when you will still be close, when you will still hold and laugh and caress each other, but in a new way, without nursing. Let them know that there will be more ways for others – brothers, sisters, Dad, friends – to be included in your loving circle.

Even though your child may not be using language yet, he or she will understand the deeper meaning of what you are saying. Remember that you are speaking to your child's "being" – their soul or natural wisdom – whether or not they give you any clear response. As you speak to them about a coming change this allows their "being" to be better prepared. Your child will hear and know that you love them, and that you take this nursing-bond seriously, and will still be there for them without nursing.

I started speaking to my son a year before we stopped nursing. I told him that during this next period of time – until he was three – we would be close and enjoy our nursing times. I gently explained that when he turned three we would explore other ways to continue being close. I asked him what his favorite snack was, and gave it to him on that special day. Our transition was easy. He took a little nibble of the treat and was done. That was it!

2. NO NEED FOR WHY. I don't believe it is necessary to explain your "Why" to your child. To burden a child with your own limitations, wants, needs or desires is too much for them. Some issues belong to the parent, and are better discussed with a partner or friend when the baby is not close by.

3. LOTS OF PLAY AND TOUCH. From the time they are born it is great to use reading or massaging or dancing or playing touch-games with your child. Then, when you start to wean, the change of that special physical closeness of nursing will not feel like a shock or a break in sharing and caring.

3. KEEP A NURSING DIARY. Writing down your thoughts and feelings about nursing and weaning is a great way to deal with questions and emotions. Record your own funny stories, insights, joys and hardships. The better you feel about yourself, and the clearer you are that it is time to complete this nursing phase, the easier it will be for your child to adjust.

Children are unique. I know some children who weaned themselves, and others who would have nursed until they were eight or nine if we let them. So, no one method will apply to every case. But one thing is important in every case: your willingness to be there for your child, through it all.

I hope this little book will serve you and your little one … and also make you smile.

Babies like to nurse, a lot —
Anytime ... anywhere ...

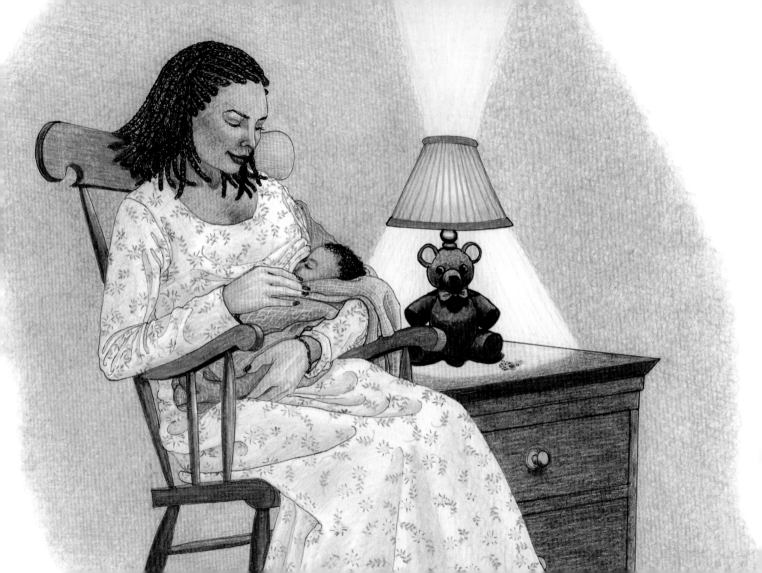

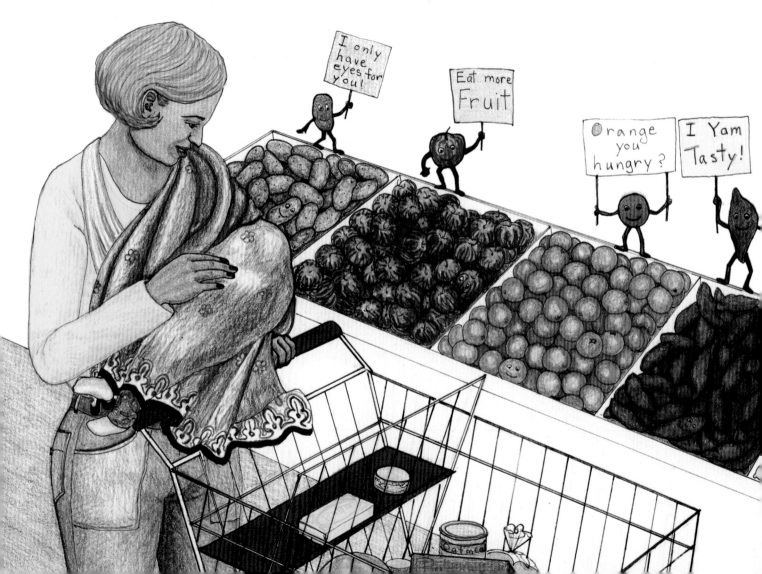

Sometimes mommies have to find unusual places that are just right for nursing.

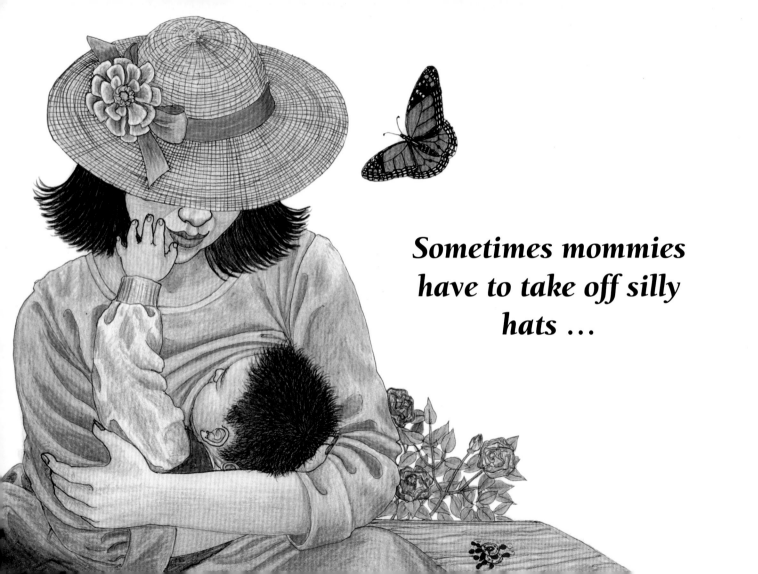

Sometimes mommies
have to take off silly
hats …

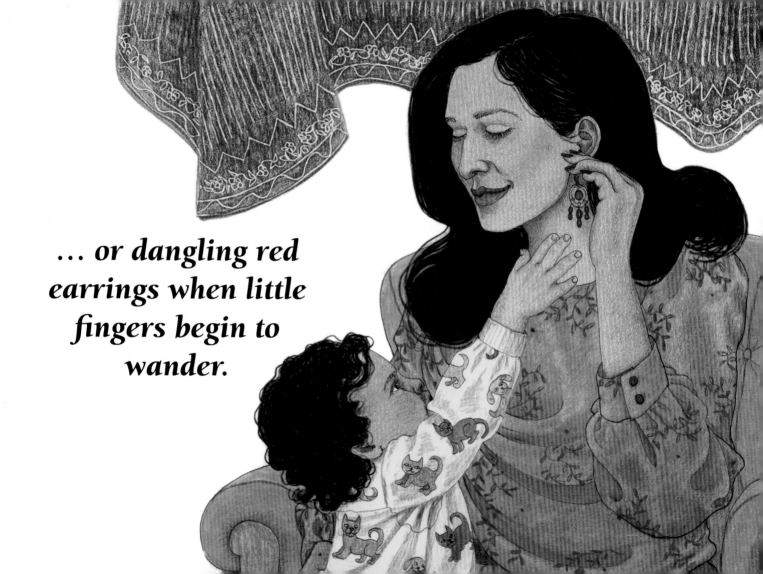

… or dangling red earrings when little fingers begin to wander.

**Mommies may have to nurse
in unusual positions.**

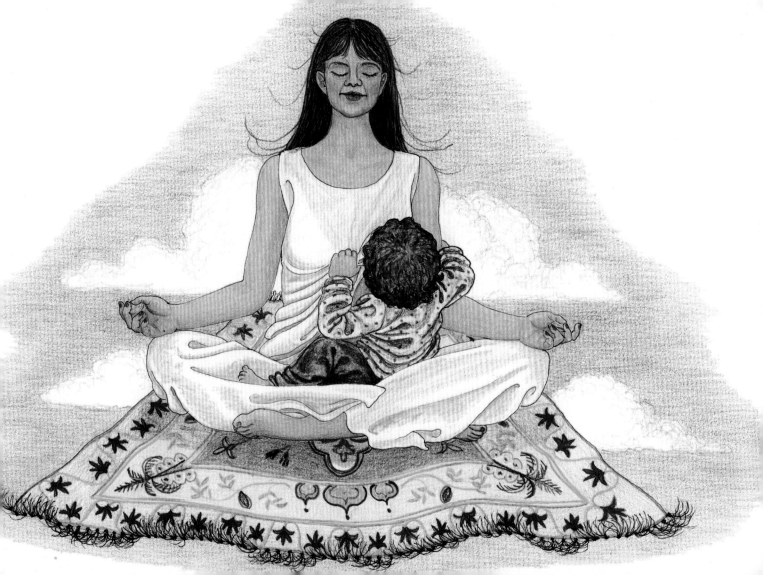

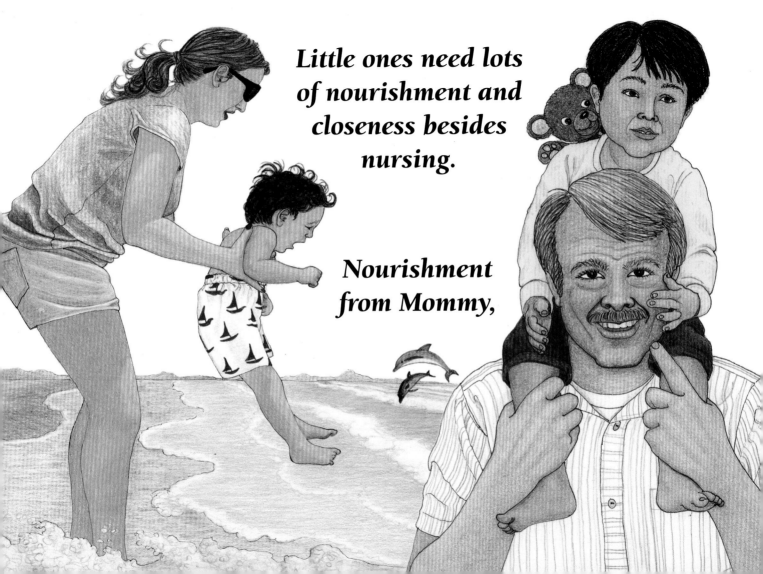

Little ones need lots of nourishment and closeness besides nursing.

Nourishment from Mommy,

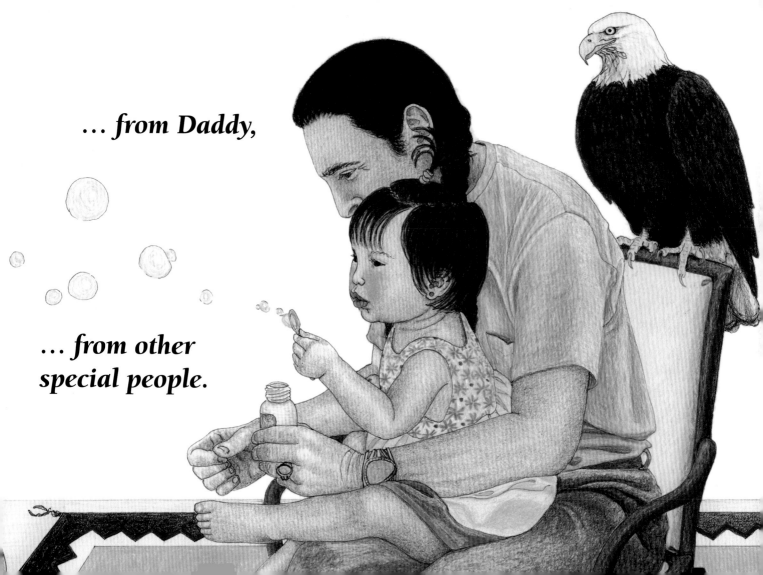

... *from Daddy,*

... *from other
special people.*

Someday, Mommy or the little one may be ready to wean. Mommy may say, "Today we will start nursing a little bit less and, when you are

_____

(fill in the blank with child's age, indicating time you will stop nursing)

"We will stop nursing and be close in other ways …

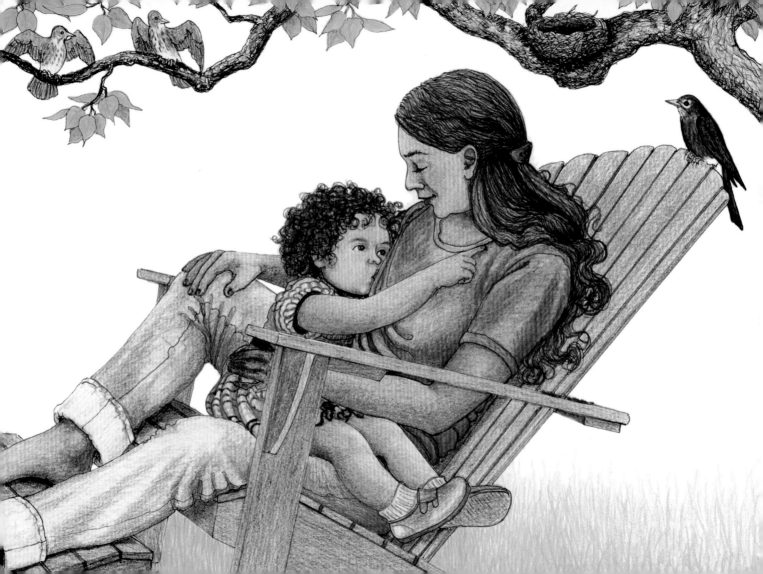

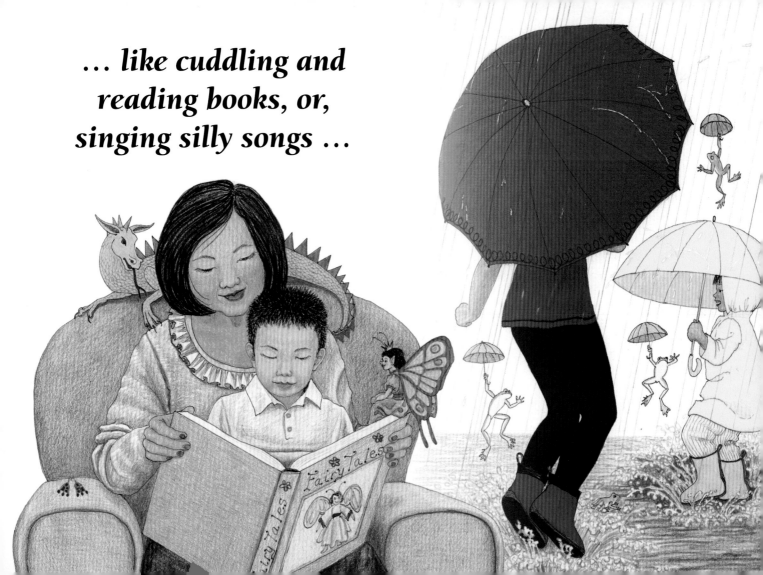

… *like cuddling and reading books, or, singing silly songs …*

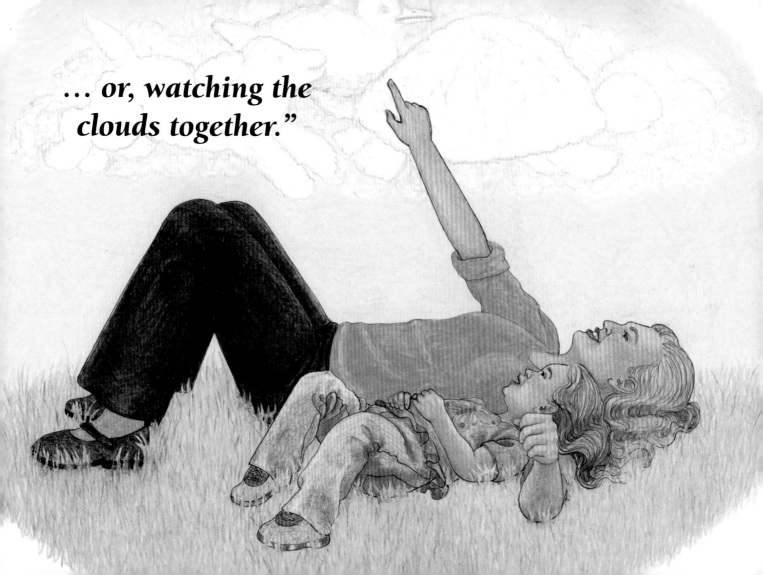

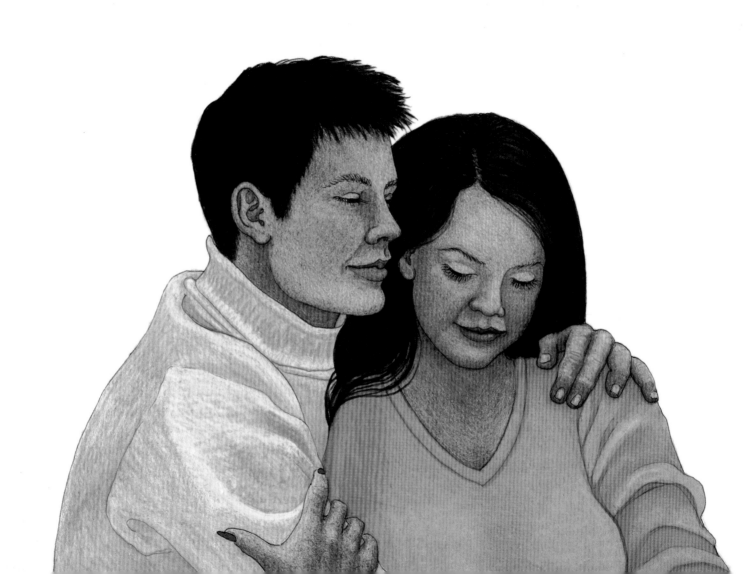

Weaning means that we are beginning to stop our breastfeeding.

How long this takes will depend on both Mommy …

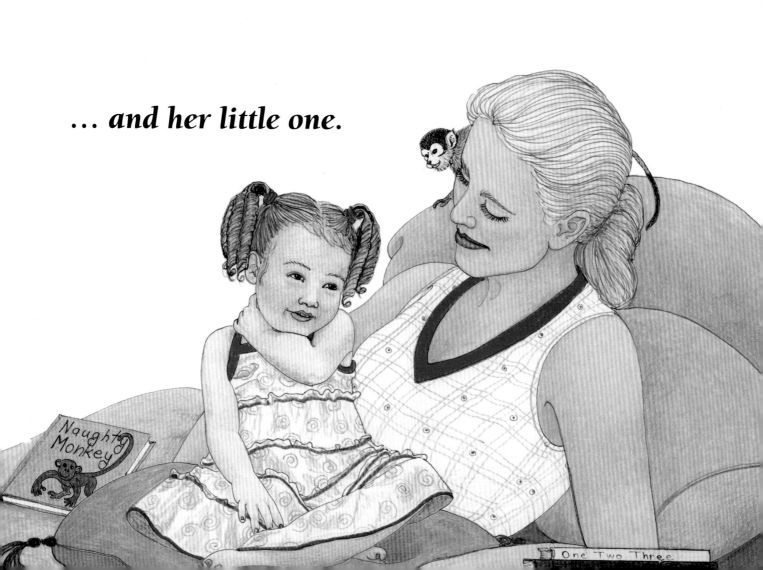

… *and her little one.*

*Mommy's milk is just the first
of many winning tastes ...*

... like juicy red strawberries floating in your cereal,

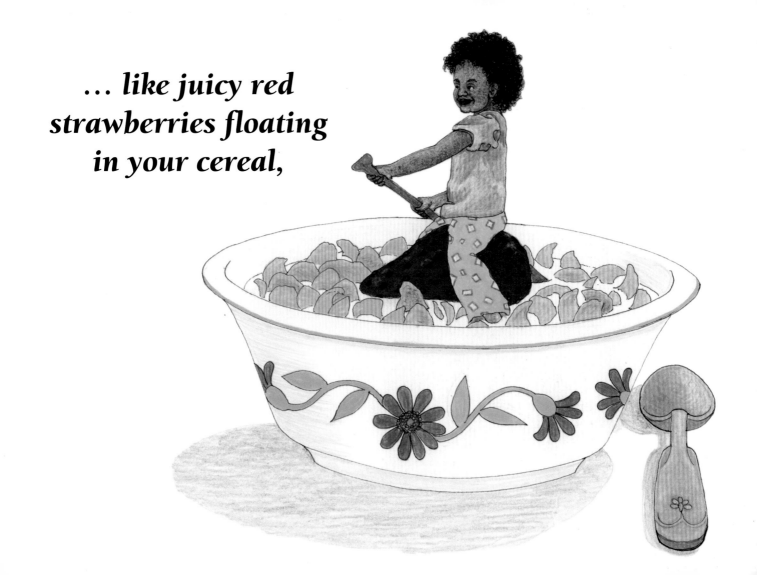

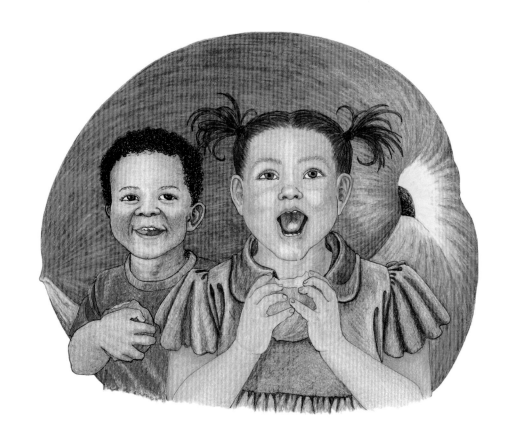

or, fresh ripe peaches dripping down your chin,

… or, crunchy carrots dipped in nut butter.

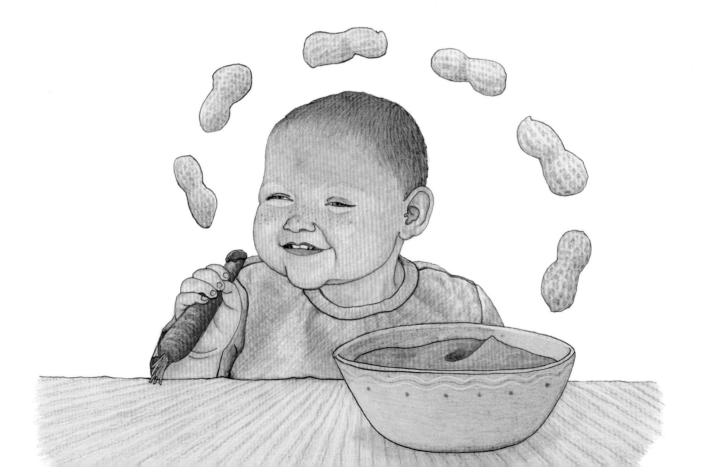

**As we grow older,
our tastes in many things change.**

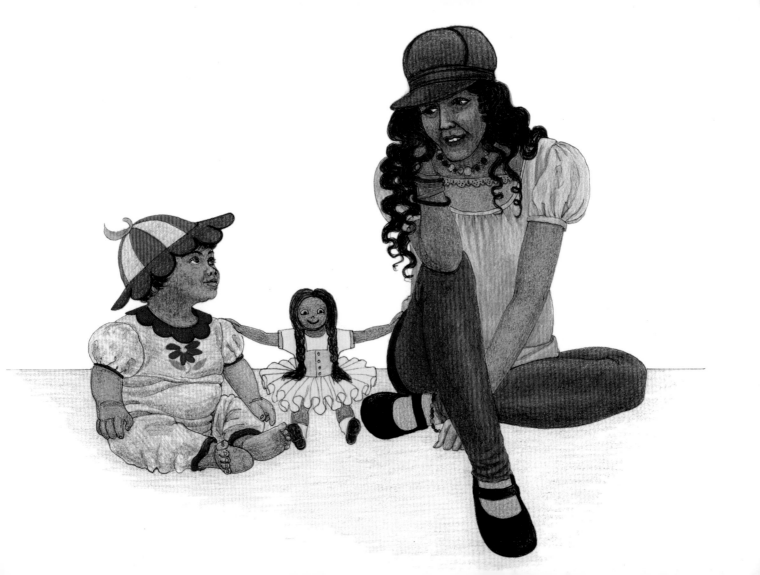

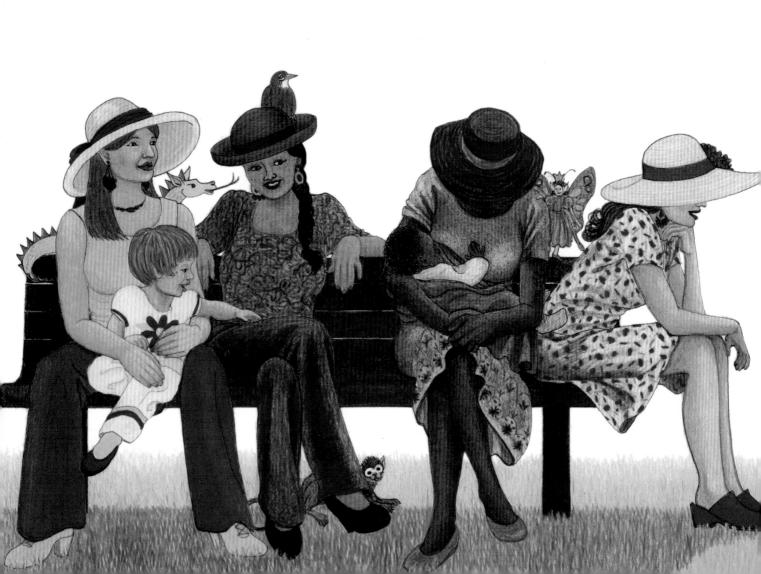

One day Mommy will wear her silly hats again ... and her dangling red earrings.

Mommy will still be close by as her little ones begin to explore the world.

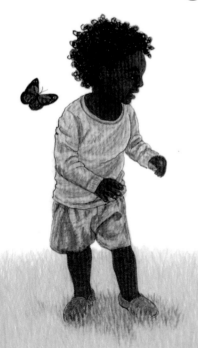

"Hey kids, wait for me!"

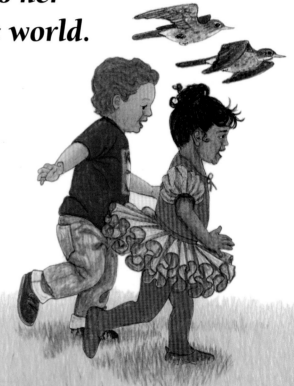

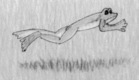

Other Titles of Interest from Kalindi Press/Hohm Press in the FAMILY HEALTH SERIES

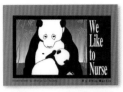

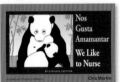

We Like To Nurse /
Nos Gusta Amamantar
by Chia Martin
Illustrations by Shukyo Rainey

English ISBN: 978-934252-45-4,
Bi-Lingual ISBN: 978-1-890772-94-9,
paper, 32 pages, $9.95

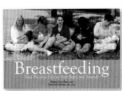

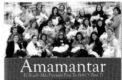

Breastfeeding / Amamantar
by Regina Sara Ryan
and Deborah Auletta, IBCLC

English ISBN: 978-1-890772-48-2,
Spanish ISBN: 978-1-890772-57-4,
paper, 32 pages, $9.95

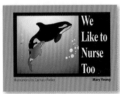

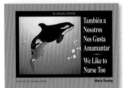

We Like to Nurse Too /
También A Nosotros Nos
Gusta Amamantar
by Mary Young

English ISBN: 978-1-890772-98-7,
Bi-Lingual ISBN: 978-1-890772-99-4,
Paper; 32 pages; $9.95

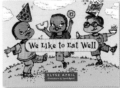

We Like to Eat Well /
Nos Gusta Comer Bien
by Elyse April
Illustrations by Lewis Agrell

English ISBN: 978-1-890772-69-7,
Bi-Lingual ISBN: 978-1-935826-01-9,
Paper; 32 pages; $9.95

TO ORDER: 1-800-381-2700 or visit our websites: www.hohmpress.com or www.kalindipress.com and click on Family Health Series. Or go directly to: www.familyhealthseries.com. Bulk Discounts Available